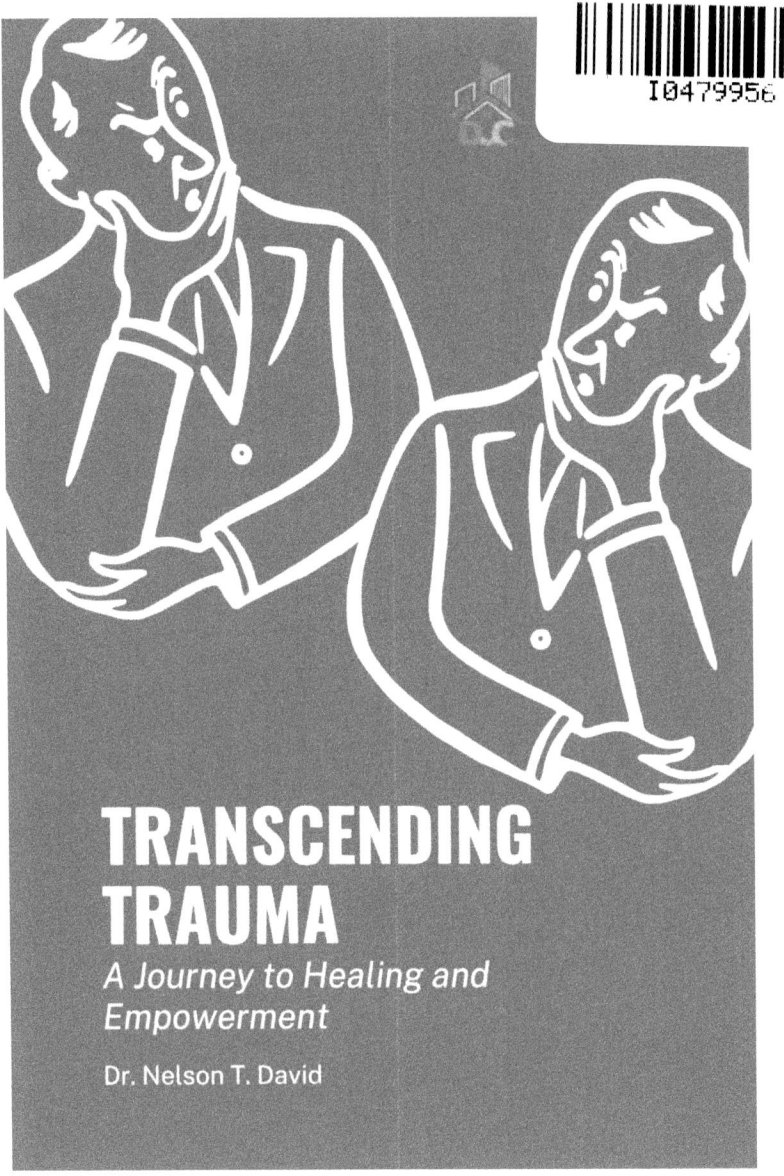

TRANSCENDING TRAUMA

A Journey to Healing and Empowerment

Dr. Nelson T. David

Foreword

Trauma is a universal experience that affects us all in different ways. It can be difficult to understand, and even harder to overcome. But it is possible. In this book, the author has taken a sensitive and compassionate approach to the topic of transcending trauma. They have delved into the various aspects of trauma, including its causes, symptoms, and effects, as well as the various coping strategies and treatments that can be used to manage it.

This book offers a holistic approach to healing, with a particular focus on self-care and self-compassion. The author has provided practical advice, as well as emotional support, for those who are struggling with trauma. They have also shared stories from individuals who have overcome their trauma, to provide hope and inspiration for readers.

I highly recommend this book to anyone who is looking for guidance and support on their journey to transcending trauma. It is a powerful and inspiring read that will leave you feeling empowered and hopeful.

Preface

Trauma is an unfortunate reality that affects many of us at some point in our lives. It can take many forms, from a one-time traumatic event to chronic, ongoing stress. The experience of trauma can be incredibly overwhelming, and the aftermath can be long-lasting. It can affect our mental and physical health, our relationships, and our ability to function in our daily lives.

This book aims to provide a comprehensive understanding of trauma, its effects, and the different ways to cope and heal from it. It's divided into five chapters that cover various aspects of trauma, including its causes, symptoms, and effects, as well as the different coping strategies and treatments that can be used to manage it. The author has also shared stories from individuals who have overcome their trauma, to provide hope and inspiration for readers.

It's important to note that this book is not a substitute for professional help, but a guide to understanding trauma and to encourage readers to seek help when they need it.

This book is written for anyone who has experienced trauma, as well as for their loved ones, friends, and mental health professionals. It's a valuable resource for anyone who is looking for guidance and support on their journey to transcending trauma.

This book is not only about understanding trauma, but also about self-care and self-compassion. It's about learning to cope with the difficult emotions and memories that come with trauma and to take steps towards healing and growth.

I hope that this book will provide valuable information and support for anyone who is struggling with trauma, and that it will inspire them to take the first step towards healing.

Acknowledgments

I would like to extend my deepest gratitude to all of the individuals who have shared their personal stories and experiences of trauma with me. Your courage and vulnerability have been an inspiration, and your contributions have made this book possible.

I would also like to thank my family and friends for their unwavering support and encouragement throughout the writing process.

I would like to express my appreciation to the professionals in the field of trauma and healing who have shared their knowledge and expertise. Your contributions have been invaluable in the creation of this book.

And finally, I would like to thank all readers, for taking the time to read this book and for being open to learning more about the topic of transcending trauma. I hope that this book has been informative and helpful for you in some way.

Introduction

1: Understanding Trauma – It defines trauma and its different types, including physical, emotional, and psychological trauma. It also explains the symptoms of trauma and how it can affect an individual's mental and physical health.

2: Coping Strategies - The chapter discusses different coping strategies that can be used to manage the symptoms of trauma, including mindfulness, journaling, and exercise. It also covers the importance of building a support system and seeking professional help.

3: Healing Trauma - The chapter covers different approaches to healing trauma, including therapy, medication, and alternative treatments. It also discusses the importance of self-care and the role of trauma in shaping an individual's identity.

4: Transcending Trauma - The chapter discusses the process of transcending trauma and the importance of forgiveness, both of oneself and others. It also covers the importance of setting goals, developing resilience, and focusing on the present.

5: Moving Forward - The chapter covers the importance of moving forward after transcending trauma and setting goals for the future. It also discusses the importance of developing resilience, learning to forgive, and understanding that healing is an ongoing process.

Overall, the book emphasizes the importance of seeking professional help, building a support system, and using coping strategies to manage the symptoms of trauma. It also covers different approaches to healing trauma and the importance of forgiveness, setting goals, and focusing on the present in order to move forward.

Table of Content

Chapter 1

Trauma

Trauma is a deeply distressing or disturbing experience that can have a significant impact on an individual's emotional, psychological, and physical well-being. Trauma can occur as a result of a single, overwhelming event, such as a natural disaster or a violent crime, or it can be the result of a series of events that occur over time, such as childhood abuse or neglect. Regardless of the cause, trauma can leave individuals feeling overwhelmed, scared, and disconnected from the world around them.

The effects of trauma can be wide-ranging and long-lasting. Some individuals may experience symptoms such as anxiety, depression, and post-traumatic stress disorder (PTSD), while others may struggle with addiction, self-harm, or other forms of self-destructive behavior. Trauma can also affect an individual's relationships, making it difficult for them to trust others or form healthy connections.

Despite the difficulties that trauma can cause, it is important to understand that healing is possible. With the right support and resources, individuals can learn to cope with their trauma and move forward with their lives. This is where the concept of "transcending trauma" comes in - it's about understanding that it is not only possible but necessary for the person to heal, be able to move on and grow from the experience.

Addressing and healing from trauma is important not only for the individual who has experienced the trauma but also for their families, friends, and communities. When individuals are able to transcend their trauma, they can become more resilient, more compassionate, and more connected to the world around them. This in turn can have a positive ripple effect on their communities, helping to create a more compassionate and understanding society as a whole.

In this Book, we will explore the different aspects of trauma, including its causes, effects, and how to heal from it. We will also discuss the different therapeutic approaches that can be used to help individuals transcend their trauma and move forward with their lives. We will also touch on the importance of self-care and building a support system in the healing process, and the concept of "post-traumatic growth" and how individuals can use their trauma to grow and improve their lives.

It's important to note that healing from trauma is a process and it can take time. It's also unique to each individual and it may require different approaches and tools. However, it is possible, and with the right support and resources, individuals can move forward and live fulfilling lives.

Chapter 2

Understanding Trauma

Trauma can take many forms, and it can be caused by a wide range of events. Some of the most common types of trauma include complex trauma, developmental trauma, and single incident trauma.

Complex trauma refers to repeated or prolonged exposure to traumatic events, often occurring in childhood. This can include experiences such as physical, sexual, or emotional abuse, neglect, or exposure to domestic violence. These types of trauma can have a significant impact on an individual's development and can affect their ability to form healthy relationships, trust others, and regulate their emotions.

Developmental trauma is similar to complex trauma but refers specifically to trauma that occurs during critical developmental periods, such as in childhood or adolescence. This type of trauma can have a significant impact on an individual's physical, emotional, and cognitive development, and can affect their ability to learn, form relationships, and regulate their emotions.

Single incident trauma refers to a traumatic event that occurs only once, such as a natural disaster, a car accident, or a violent crime. While the impact of this type of trauma can be severe, it is often more short-lived than complex or developmental trauma.

Regardless of the type of trauma, individuals who have experienced it may experience a wide range of symptoms. Some of the most common symptoms of trauma include:

- ❖ Intrusive thoughts or memories of the traumatic event

- ❖ Avoidance of reminders of the traumatic event

- ❖ Hyper vigilance or an exaggerated startle response

- ❖ Anxiety, depression, or other mood disorders

- ❖ Difficulty sleeping or nightmares

- ❖ Difficulty trusting others or forming relationships

- ❖ Anger, irritability, or agitation

- ❖ Flashbacks or dissociation

❖ Physical symptoms such as headaches, stomach pain, or muscle tension

It's important to note that everyone responds differently to trauma and the symptoms may vary depending on the individual and the type of trauma. Additionally, the symptoms may not always be apparent immediately after the traumatic event and may appear later on.

It's also worth mentioning the concept of "trauma-informed care" which is an approach that acknowledges the prevalence of trauma and its impact on individuals and communities, and aims to create a safe and healing environment for those who have experienced trauma. This approach is used in various fields such as healthcare, education, and social services. It involves understanding how trauma can affect an individual's behavior and interactions, and being responsive to the needs of that person, providing them with the necessary support and resources to heal.

We have explored the different types of trauma and the symptoms that individuals who have experienced trauma may experience. In the following chapters, we will discuss the therapeutic approaches that can be used to help individuals heal from trauma and transcend it.

It's important to remember that healing from trauma is a process that requires time, patience, and the right support. With the right resources and guidance, individuals can learn to cope with their trauma and move forward with their lives.

Chapter 3

Therapeutic Approaches for Transcending Trauma

There are a variety of therapeutic approaches that can be used to help individuals heal from trauma and transcend it. These approaches can include both traditional and alternative methods, and may involve working with a therapist or other healthcare professional.

One of the most commonly used therapeutic approaches for trauma is cognitive-behavioral therapy (CBT). This approach focuses on helping individuals identify and change negative thought patterns and behaviors that may be contributing to their symptoms. CBT can be used to address a wide range of symptoms, including anxiety, depression, and post-traumatic stress disorder (PTSD).

Another commonly used therapeutic approach is eye movement desensitization and reprocessing (EMDR). EMDR is a form of therapy that uses bilateral stimulation, such as eye movements, sounds, or taps, to help process and integrate traumatic memories. EMDR can be particularly effective for individuals who are experiencing symptoms of PTSD.

Another approach is called somatic therapy, it's a form of therapy that focuses on the body and the connection between the mind and the body. This approach can help individuals to understand and process their trauma by exploring the physical sensations and emotions that are associated with it. This type of therapy can be beneficial for individuals who may have difficulty expressing themselves verbally or have difficulty processing their trauma through traditional talk therapy.

For some, incorporating mindfulness practices such as yoga, meditation, and body-based therapies like dance or movement therapy, can also be helpful in the healing process. These practices can help individuals to increase their awareness of the present moment, reduce symptoms of anxiety and depression, and improve their overall well-being.

Art therapy is another approach that can be beneficial for individuals who have experienced trauma. This type of therapy allows individuals to express themselves through art and can help them to process and understand their trauma in a non-verbal way.

It's important to note that these are just a few examples of the many therapeutic approaches that can be used to help individuals transcend their trauma. The approach that will be most effective will depend on the individual, the type of trauma they have experienced, and the symptoms they are experiencing. It's also worth mentioning that seeking a professional help is important, in order to get the right guidance and assessment to determine the best course of action.

In addition to seeking professional help, it's also important to build a support system, which can include friends, family, and loved ones. Supportive people can provide emotional support, validation, and understanding, which can be crucial in the healing process.

We discussed therapeutic approaches that can be used to help individuals transcend their trauma. From traditional talk therapy to alternative methods, there are many different options available to help individuals heal. It's important to remember that healing from trauma is a process that requires time, patience, and the right support. With the help of a professional, and with the support of loved ones, individuals can learn to cope with their trauma and move forward with their lives.

Chapter 4

Coping Strategies for Transcending Trauma

In addition to seeking professional help and building a support system, there are also a variety of coping strategies that individuals can use to help them transcend their trauma. These strategies can be used in conjunction with therapeutic approaches to help individuals better manage their symptoms and improve their overall well-being.

One important coping strategy is self-care. This can include taking care of physical needs, such as getting enough sleep, eating a healthy diet, and engaging in regular physical activity. It can also include practicing relaxation techniques, such as deep breathing, meditation, or yoga, to help manage stress and anxiety.

Another important coping strategy is journaling. Writing about one's thoughts and feelings can be a helpful way to process and understand them. It can also be a useful tool for identifying negative thought patterns and behaviors that may be contributing to symptoms.

Another coping strategy is social support, which can be provided by friends, family, or support groups. Supportive people can provide emotional support, validation, and understanding, which can be crucial in the healing process. Joining a support group can also provide individuals with the opportunity to connect with others who have experienced similar trauma, which can help them to feel less alone and more understood.

Another strategy is to focus on mindfulness, which is the practice of being present in the moment. Mindfulness can help individuals to focus on the present moment and let go of negative thoughts and feelings about the past or future. It can also help individuals to reduce stress and improve their overall well-being.

Another coping strategy is to engage in creative activities, such as painting, drawing, or writing. These activities can provide a healthy outlet for emotions and help individuals to process and understand their trauma in a non-verbal way.

It's important to note that these are just a few examples of the many coping strategies that can be used to help individuals transcend their trauma. The strategies that will be most effective will depend on the individual, the type of trauma they have experienced, and the symptoms they are experiencing. It's also important to remember that coping strategies are not a replacement for professional help, they are tools that can be used in conjunction with therapy to help individuals better manage their symptoms and improve their overall well-being.

Another important aspect of coping with trauma is learning how to manage triggers, which are events or situations that can cause individuals to relive their traumatic experience. Triggers can include certain sights, sounds, smells, or even certain emotions. When individuals are triggered, they may experience feelings of anxiety, fear, or even panic. It's important for individuals to be aware of their triggers and have a plan in place for managing them.

Lastly, it's important to understand that healing from trauma is a process, and it may not happen overnight. It's important to be patient with oneself and understand that progress may be slow. It's also important to remember that setbacks are a normal part of the healing process. Coping strategies and therapeutic approaches can help individuals to manage their symptoms and improve their overall well-being, but it takes time and effort.

Variety of coping strategies that can be used to help individuals transcend their trauma. From self-care to social support, there are many different options available to help individuals better manage their symptoms and improve their overall well-being. It's important to remember that healing from trauma is a process that requires time, patience, and the right support. With the help of a professional, and with the support of loved ones, individuals can learn to cope with their trauma and move forward with their lives.

Chapter 5

Moving Forward After Transcending Trauma

Transcending trauma is a journey, and the process of healing can take time. However, with the help of professional help, coping strategies, and a strong support system, individuals can learn to manage their symptoms and improve their overall well-being. Once an individual has made progress in dealing with their trauma, they may be ready to begin thinking about moving forward with their life.

One important aspect of moving forward is setting goals. Setting goals can help individuals to focus on the future and give them a sense of purpose. These goals can be small or big and can be related to any area of life such as career, education, relationships, and personal growth. Setting goals can provide a sense of direction and motivation and can help individuals to feel a sense of control over their lives.

Another important aspect of moving forward is developing a sense of resilience. Resilience is the ability to bounce back from difficult situations and is an essential component of mental well-being. Individuals who have experienced trauma may have a harder time developing resilience, but it is possible to learn how to do so. Building resilience can involve learning new coping strategies, developing a support system, and learning to reframe negative thoughts.

Another aspect is to learn to forgive, both oneself and others. Forgiving oneself for what happened during the trauma can be difficult, but it is an important step in the healing process. Forgiving others who may have caused the trauma can also be difficult, but it can help to let go of anger and resentment and move forward.

Another important step is to learn how to live in the present. Trauma can make it difficult to focus on the present and enjoy life, but it is important to learn how to do so. Engaging in activities that bring joy, such as hobbies, spending time with loved ones, and traveling can help individuals to focus on the present and enjoy life.

Lastly, it's important to understand that healing from trauma is ongoing process and that individuals may experience setbacks. It's important to have a plan in place for dealing with setbacks and to understand that they are a normal part of the healing process.

We have discussed the importance of setting goals, developing resilience, learning to forgive, living in the present and understanding that healing is an ongoing process. As individuals continue to make progress in managing their trauma, they can begin to think about moving forward with their lives. It's important to remember that healing is a journey and that setbacks are a normal part of the process. With the help of professional help, coping strategies, and a strong support system, individuals can learn to manage their symptoms and improve their overall well-being.

Transcending trauma is a difficult process, but it is possible. It's important to seek professional help, build a support system, and use coping strategies to manage symptoms. It's also important to set goals, develop resilience, learn to forgive, and focus on the present. Remember that healing from trauma is a journey and that setbacks are a normal part of the process. With time, patience, and the right support, individuals can learn to cope with their trauma and move forward with their lives.

Conclusion

Transcending Trauma: A Journey to Healing and Empowerment" is an essential resource for anyone who has experienced trauma. The author expertly covers the topic of trauma and provides a thorough understanding of its effects and the different coping strategies and treatments available. The book offers hope and inspiration for those on their journey to healing, and emphasizes the importance of seeking professional help. The author's compassionate approach and professional expertise make this book a trustworthy and valuable guide for anyone seeking to understand and transcending their trauma.

Note: *Encourage readers to seek help if they are struggling with trauma and remind them that healing is possible.*

It's important to remember that if you are struggling with trauma, you are not alone. Trauma is a common experience and healing is possible. Seeking professional help, building a support system, and using coping strategies can all be effective ways to manage the symptoms of trauma and begin the healing process.

Don't be afraid to reach out for help. Whether it's talking to a therapist, counselor, or support group, there are many resources available to help individuals who have experienced trauma. These professionals can provide guidance and support as you navigate the healing process. They can also help you develop a personalized plan for coping with your trauma and moving forward with your life.

It is important to remember that healing is not a quick or easy process, but it is possible. You may have setbacks and difficult days, but it is important to keep moving forward and know that healing is possible. It takes time, patience, and the right support, but with the right tools, you can learn to cope with your trauma and live a fulfilling life.

In short, if you are struggling with trauma, know that you are not alone and that healing is possible. Don't be afraid to reach out for help and remember that professional help, support system and coping strategies can be effective ways to manage symptoms and begin the healing process. It's important to remember that healing is a journey, and that setbacks are a normal part of the process. Be patient with yourself and keep moving forward, know that healing is possible.

Offer hope and inspiration for readers who are working towards transcending their trauma.

It's important to remember that transcending trauma is a journey, and it takes time and effort, but it is possible. The road to healing may be long, but it is worth it. The process of transcending trauma can be challenging, but it can also be incredibly rewarding. As you work towards healing, you will learn new skills, gain insight into yourself, and build resilience.

You are not alone in your journey, and it's important to surround yourself with supportive people who understand what you're going through and can offer encouragement and understanding. Remember to be kind to yourself, and don't be afraid to ask for help when you need it.

As you work towards transcending your trauma, it's important to focus on the present and take things one day at a time. Set small, achievable goals for yourself, and celebrate your accomplishments as you achieve them.

Remember that healing is not a linear process, and it's normal to have setbacks along the way. Be patient with yourself and know that it's okay to take a step back when you need to.

Above all, know that you are strong and capable of healing. You have already overcome so much, and you will continue to do so. Keep pushing forward, and don't give up hope. You deserve to live a happy, healthy, and fulfilling life, and you can get there.

In summary, transcending trauma is a journey, and it takes time and effort, but it is possible. Remember to surround yourself with supportive people, be kind to yourself, focus on the present, set small achievable goals, and don't give up hope. You are strong and capable of healing. Keep pushing forward, and you will get there.

www.ingramcontent.com/pod-product-compliance
Lightning Source LLC
Chambersburg PA
CBHW070752220526
45467CB00018B/2071